Information Circular 9473

Drill Rig Incident

By Edward A. Barrett and Roberta A. Calhoun

U.S. DEPARTMENT OF HEALTH AND HUMAN SERVICES
Centers for Disease Control and Prevention
National Institute for Occupational Safety and Health
Pittsburgh Research Laboratory
Pittsburgh, PA

February 2005

ORDERING INFORMATION

Copies of National Institute for Occupational Safety and Health (NIOSH)
documents and information
about occupational safety and health are available from

NIOSH–Publications Dissemination
4676 Columbia Parkway
Cincinnati, OH 45226–1998

FAX 513–533–8573
Telephone: 1–800–35–NIOSH
(1–800–356–4674)
E-mail: pubstaff@cdc.gov
Web site: www.cdc.gov/niosh

DHHS (NIOSH) Publication No. 2005–108

Table of Contents

Appendices

    Appendix A: Problem booklet (duplicate this copy for use in class)

    Appendix B: Blank answer sheets (print the invisible ink answers on this)

    Appendix C: Invisible ink answers (print these on the answer sheet)

    Appendix D: Pretest / posttest questions

DRILL RIG INCIDENT

By Edward A. Barrett[1] and Roberta A. Calhoun[2]

Introduction

This Instructor's Copy contains most of the materials trainers will need in order to use Drill Rig Incident (DRI). It includes suggestions for using the exercise, performance objectives for the training, master answer sheets, a scoring key, and a set of discussion notes that provides additional subject information. Four appendices are also included. Appendix A is the complete exercise problem booklet. It may be reproduced so that every person in the training class has one. Appendix B contains answer sheet blanks. The blanks are furnished if you choose to have the invisible ink answers that appear in appendix C printed on them at your location.[3] Answer sheets are consumable. One is needed for each group of three to five persons who work the exercise together. An alternative is for each individual trainee to have his/her own answer sheet. Appendix D contains the 24-question pretest / posttest that was used in the field evaluation of the DRI exercise.

Acknowledgment

The authors thank Linda J. McWilliams, Statistician, NIOSH Pittsburgh Research Laboratory, for her assistance in analyzing the experimental data in this document.

---

[1]Mining engineer.
[2]Safety and occupational health specialist.
Pittsburgh Research Laboratory, National Institute for Occupational Safety and Health, Pittsburgh, PA.
[3]You can do this yourself if you have the proper equipment, or you can contact a local printer.

Exercise Summary

The following summary information is provided to help you decide if this exercise is appropriate for your training class.

<u>Type</u>:   Invisible ink

<u>Length</u>:   Eleven questions (20 minutes for administration plus varying times for followup discussion)

<u>Skills</u>:   Recognizing basic facts about noise, hearing loss, and hearing protection
Identifying ways to protect hearing
Wearing hearing protection properly

<u>Location</u>:   Surface drill site

<u>Problem</u>:   You are the drill crew foreman. At the beginning of the day shift, your helper latches the breakout wrench around the first pipe section as you begin to remove rod sections from a drill hole. Your helper is supposed to step back at this point in case the wire rope holding the wrench should break. He doesn't step back on his own and also fails to respond to you shouting at him to step back. In a split second, you must decide what to do.

There is a related training exercise available entitled *Wearing Hearing Protection Properly: A 3-D Training Aid for Drillers*, DHHS (NIOSH) Publication No. 2005–107 (IC 9472). It can be obtained by contacting NIOSH at:

Telephone: 1–800–35–NIOSH (1–800–356–4674)
Fax: 513–533–8573
E-mail: pubstaff@cdc.gov
www.cdc.gov/niosh

How to Use the Exercise

1. Look at the performance objectives on the next page. Decide if the exercise is appropriate for your training needs.

2. Work through the exercise using the developing pen and score your responses.

3. Review the master answer sheet. Look at all of the answers, both correct and incorrect.

4. Study the Instructor's Discussion Notes for the exercise.

5. Become thoroughly familiar with the problem so that you can present it to your class without reading it.

6. When you present the exercise to your class:

    •   Give each person an exercise problem booklet, and give each group of three to five persons an answer sheet and a developing pen.[4]

    •   Go over the instructions for the exercise.

    •   Demonstrate how to select and mark answers using the developing pen.

    •   Explain the problem, making sure that everyone understands the situation.

    •   Have the class work the exercise.

    •   When class members finish, ask them to figure their scores using the instructions at the end of the exercise.

    •   After everyone in the class has finished, review the exercise. Discuss why certain answers are correct and why others are incorrect.[5] Add your own ideas.

---

[4]An alternative would be to give each person in the class an answer sheet and developing pen in addition to the problem booklet.

[5]Regardless of whether the exercise is completed by a small group of trainees or an individual, class discussion is an important followup to the training.

Performance Objectives

Objective Number	Capability Verb(s)	Description of required performance and conditions under which it is to occur
1. DR[6]	Recall Apply	The initial action in the event of an emergency should always be to shut down the rig using a kill switch
2. HL	Recall	Basic facts about individual hearing loss
3. HL	Recognize	The signs that workers should use to determine if they have a hearing loss
4. HL	Recall	The personal and job-related benefits of protecting the hearing that workers have left
5. N	Identify	Conditions in the workplace indicating that surrounding noise levels are too loud
6. N	Apply	Procedures and practices that may be used to deal with loud noise coming from drill rigs
7. HP	Recall Apply	Procedures for wearing hearing protection properly

---

[6]Skill and knowledge domain abbreviations:
    DR = Drill rig safety
    HL = Hearing loss
    HP = Hearing protection
    N = Noise

Master Answer Sheet for *Drill Rig Incident*

Use this answer sheet to mark your selections. Rub the developing pen gently and smoothly between the brackets. Don't scrub the pen or the message may blur. Be sure to color in the entire message once you have made a selection, otherwise you may not get all the information you need. The last part of the message will tell you what to do next.

Question A (Choose only ONE unless you are told to "Try again.")

1. [This is not the first thing that needs to be done. Try again.   ]

2. [This is not the first thing that needs to be done. Besides, you don't want to   ]
    [cause Vinny to look away from the drill. Try again.   ]

3. [You know that wire ropes have been known to snap. You should do   ]
    [something now. Try again.   ]

4. [Correct. You need to stop the rig before Vinny gets hurt. Do the next   ]
    [question.   ]

Question B (Choose only ONE unless you are told to "Try again.")

5. [There was no apparent injury, but for Vinny's sake something should be   ]
    [done. Try again.   ]

6. [This isn't important right now. You will probably learn why the rope broke   ]
    [later on. Try again.   ]

7. [Correct. For Vinny's protection in case any medical problems develop later,   ]
    [the safety manager will need to have some record of the incident. Do the   ]
    [next question.   ]

8. [Finding someone to blame is not important. Try again.   ]

9. [You need to do something else first. Try again.   ]

Question C (Select as MANY as you think are correct.)

10. [Finding someone to blame isn't going to help the situation.   ]

11. [Correct. Since no one got hurt he wants to learn the details before anyone   ]
     [forgets what happened.   ]

12. [Correct. He may be able to prevent similar incidents by developing SOPs   ]
     [and safety or toolbox meetings using this information.   ]

13. [Correct. It is often possible to develop safer ways to complete a task by   ]
     [looking at details of previous incidents.   ]

Question D (Select as MANY as you think are correct.)

14. [Even though the weather was foggy, the distance between you and Vinny   ]
    [was so close that visibility was not a problem.   ]

15. [Correct. The usual work practice is for your helper to back away as soon]
    [as he puts the wrench on a rod section.   ]

16. [Correct. This is an obvious factor that led to the incident.   ]

17. [Correct. He stayed there because he didn't follow your directions to move]
    [back.   ]

18. [Even though drill rigs are noisy, Vinny should have been able to hear your]
    [directions.   ]

Question E (Choose only ONE unless you are told to "Try again.")

19. [Vinny would have been able to hear you shouting even if he was wearing foam]
    [ear plugs. Try again.   ]

20. [Vinny knows the dangers in drilling, so he was probably paying very close]
    [attention. Try again.   ]

21. [Vinny has enough experience around drill rigs to know that wire ropes can]
    [break. Try again.   ]

22. [Correct. If Vinny has a hearing loss, this would explain why he didn't hear your]
    [original instructions or your shouting. Do the next question.   ]

Question F (Select as MANY as you think are correct.)

23. [Correct. Once your hearing is lost, it will never come back.   ]

24. [Our ears don't adjust to loud noise; we just lose our ability to hear normal]
    [sounds.   ]

25. [Correct. Damage to a person's hearing cannot be reversed.   ]

26. [Correct. There are a number of things a person can do to prevent   ]
    [hearing loss.   ]

27. [There is no way to "cure" hearing loss. Hearing aids can help some people,]
    [but not everyone can be helped by a hearing aid.   ]

28. [Correct. Stress can develop in persons who have lost some of their hearing]
    [because communication becomes difficult.   ]

29. [Permanent hearing loss can develop very quickly if noise levels are high.]

Question G (Select as MANY as you think are correct.)

30. [Correct. If this happens most of the time, it's one sign that a person may]
     [have a hearing loss.]

31. [This doesn't necessarily mean that they have a hearing problem. A loud]
     [voice may be normal for some people.]

32. [Correct. In most cases, this indicates a hearing loss.]

33. [Correct. With a hearing loss, it is difficult to hear all of the sounds that are]
     [spoken. Conversation may sound like people are mumbling.]

34. [Correct. Called tinnitus, this is a classic symptom of hearing loss.]

35. [Correct.]

Question H (Select as MANY as you think are correct.)

36. [Correct. Loud noise often causes physical pain in a person's ears.]

37. [Correct. Some call this the "2-foot rule," and it's a good way for drillers and]
     [other workers to realize that noise in their workplace is too loud.]

38. [Correct. Noise is too loud if you can't hear someone talking from 2 feet]
     [away.]

Question I (Select as MANY as you think are correct.)

39. [This will not contribute to noise reduction.]

40. [Correct. Getting away from drill rig noise for short periods of time will help to]
     [reduce their total exposure time during a shift.]

41. [Correct. It's possible that some type of control can be used to reduce]
     [drill rig noise levels or time of worker exposure to noise.]

42. [Correct. This is a sure way to protect a person's hearing.]

43. [Noise from other equipment just adds to the total noise level and would only]
     [make matters worse.]

44. [Correct. This is a reminder to all workers that noise levels are high and that]
     [everyone should be using hearing protection.]

Question J (Select as MANY as you think are correct.)

45. [Correct. Any growth of beard or sideburns will affect the seal and is   ]
     [discouraged.   ]

46. [Correct. This makes the ear plugs thinner so they can be inserted into   ]
     [your ear canal.   ]

47. [Correct. This will straighten out the ear canal and make it easier to insert   ]
     [the plug.   ]

48. [You need to use your finger to keep it in place in the ear canal while it   ]
     [swells up.   ]

49. [Correct. Combining both types of hearing protection should be done <u>only</u> for]
     [very loud noise.   ]

50. [Dirty ear plugs do not give the same protection as clean ones. There is   ]
     [also a danger of infection. Dirty ear plugs should be thrown away and   ]
     [replaced with new ones.   ]

Question K (Select as MANY as you think are correct.)

51. [Correct.   ]

52. [Correct.   ]

53. [Correct.   ]

54. [Correct. Although hearing aids may help, they can never bring back   ]
     [normal hearing.   ]

Finding your score

Number of "Correct" answers you colored in   = (1) _____

21 minus number of incorrect answers you colored in   = (2) _____

Add (1) and (2) to get your total score   = (3) _____

Highest possible score = 54

Lowest possible score = 0

Instructor's Discussion Notes

General Information

Use the information presented here, along with your own ideas, to discuss the exercise with the class after it is completed. Group discussion will help strengthen knowledge and skills learned by relating the subject material in the exercise to the background and experiences of workers. Trainees generally enjoy discussing the answers, and in doing so, they often suggest other appropriate responses based on their experience. The purpose of *Drill Rig Incident* is to teach workers about noise, hearing loss, and hearing protection. Reviewing answers can contribute to this goal by focusing on the interests and needs of trainees.

It is often helpful to review the exercise by showing overhead transparencies of all answers while workers follow along in their problem booklets. This allows you to lead the group through the exercise and to discuss both correct and incorrect responses to each question. Overheads of all answers can be made using the master answer sheets, which begin on page 5.

The following discussion notes provide additional information for your use. Read through and think about the notes before the training class. Incorporate the information you find here with your own knowledge, and make these points at the appropriate places in the followup discussions.

Special Emphasis Questions

After field tests were completed in the evaluation phase of *Drill Rig Incident*, it was noted that of the 54 total responses to the 11 questions (A through K), 6 were incorrectly identified by a high percentage of trainees. One of the six is a correct answer that should have been revealed using the developing pen, but was not. The other five are incorrect answers that should not have been revealed, but were. It is recommended that the instructor place additional emphasis on these six responses during class discussions. Additional information is provided for this purpose in the next section.

Question D
18. Loud drill rig noise.
    [Even though drill rigs are noisy, Vinny should have been able to hear your   ]
    [directions.   ]

Question E
20. Vinny wasn't paying attention.
    [Vinny knows the dangers in drilling, so he was probably paying very close   ]
    [attention. Try again.   ]

Question F

29. Hearing loss develops after many years of exposure to loud noise.
     [Permanent hearing loss can develop very quickly if noise levels are high.   ]

Question G

31. Someone tells them they talk too loud.
     [This doesn't necessarily mean that they have a hearing problem. A loud   ]
     [voice may be normal for some people.   ]

Question J

45. Keep beards or long sideburns trimmed so they don't affect the seal of earmuffs.
     [Correct. Any growth of beard or sideburns will affect the seal and is   ]
     [discouraged.   ]

48. After placing the rolled and squeezed ear plug in your ear, release it. It will expand
     to give you a snug fit.
     [You need to use your finger to keep it in place in the ear canal while it   ]
     [swells up.   ]

Discussion

Question A – The correct answer is 4. The best action to take at this point is to hit a kill switch. The wire rope holding a wrench can break. According to the Occupational Safety and Health Administration (OSHA), a fatality occurred in 1989 when a worker was hit by a drill rig pipe tong (wrench) handle that rotated freely after the wire rope, to which it was attached, snapped. An OSHA investigation found that one of the factors causing the incident was that the wire rope snub line was too long. Workers around a drill rig must know where kill switches are located and not hesitate to use them in case of an emergency.

Question B – The correct answer is 7. Most of the test subjects answered this question correctly. It is wise, and very often company policy, to inform someone responsible for employee safety as soon as possible after an incident occurs.

Question C – The correct answers are 11, 12, and 13. All of these are reasons that a safety manager should talk with workers after an incident. Gathering information from those involved will generally yield valuable insight that can be used in a variety of constructive ways. Workers should be reminded that a safety manager's function is not to lay blame. Pointing a finger doesn't solve problems. At this point, he doesn't know what the problem is, and it is his responsibility to find out.

Question D – The correct answers are 15, 16, and 17. These are somewhat common factors that contribute to many workplace incidents, and they clearly played a role here. It was stated in the background information that the weather is cool and foggy; however, the driller and helper generally work in such close proximity that one would not expect fog to be a problem (14).

More than two-thirds of the test subjects also chose 18 as one of the correct responses:
18.   Loud drill rig noise.
      [Even though drill rigs are noisy, Vinny should have been able to hear your   ]
      [directions.   ]
A common practice at drill sites is to communicate by shouting above the noise produced by running equipment, in this case a drill rig. Loud noise is routine and therefore should not be considered a factor contributing to Vinny's incident.

Question E – The correct answer is 22. Two things occurred early on that indicate the communication breakdown between the driller and Vinny could have been due to Vinny's hearing loss. Vinny was reminded by his driller to "step back after you attach the automatic chuck," and after he latched the breakout wrench around the first pipe section, his driller shouted the word "back" to him. Vinny, an experienced drill rig worker, didn't heed either warning because he didn't hear them. Vinny wasn't wearing any type of hearing protection and, even if he had been using foam ear plugs, he still should have been able to hear someone shouting at him (19).

More than half of the test subjects chose 20 as the correct answer:
20.   Vinny wasn't paying attention.
      [Vinny knows the dangers in drilling, so he was probably paying very close   ]
      [attention. Try again.   ]
Because Vinny has 5 years of experience on a drill crew, he was probably paying close attention to what he was doing. Also, because of his experience, it is likely that Vinny is aware that wire ropes holding a breakout wrench can snap (21).

Question F – The correct answers are 23, 25, 26, and 28. Hearing loss is permanent (23). Exposure to loud noise can result in what may seem to be a temporary loss of hearing. Even though hearing seems to return to "normal" after a brief period of time, some small loss actually occurs. Loud noise damages the hair cells and nerves in the inner ear, which cannot be replaced or repaired. Exposure to multiple short, loud noises adds up and eventually results in permanent damage, similar to what happens from continuous exposure.

The understanding that hearing loss is permanent is the main reason to protect hearing at all times, both at the workplace and away from it. Hearing loss is preventable (26). Even if some hearing has been lost, the remaining hearing needs to be protected. Some hearing is better than none at all. Once hearing is lost, it is gone forever and cannot be reversed (25). There is no known way to "cure" hearing loss (27). Damaged hair cells and nerves cannot be repaired and returned to normal.

Our ears never adjust to loud noise (24). It may seem that a noise doesn't sound quite as loud as it once did, but this is because some of our ability to hear it has been lost, not because our ears have adjusted to it.

Hearing loss can result in stress. This is one of the consequences of hearing loss that is not well-known. People with a hearing loss develop stress because of their inability to hear some, or all, of what others are saying.

More than half of the test subjects chose 29 as a correct answer:
29.   Hearing loss develops after many years of exposure to loud noise.
       [Permanent hearing loss can develop very quickly if noise levels are high.   ]
Trainees should be reminded that (1) loud noise can damage the ears instantly, (2) continuous exposures can cause a similar hearing loss over a period of time, and (3) age has nothing to do with (1) or (2).

Question G – The correct answers are 30, 32, 33, 34, and 35. It is important for workers to be able to assess their own level of hearing. They are more likely to protect the hearing they have left when they know and accept the fact that some of their hearing is gone. Workers need to be aware that one sign of a hearing loss is asking others to repeat what has been said (30). Problems hearing normal conversation (32), complaints about people mumbling (33), and turning up the TV volume (35) are also signs of hearing loss. Constant buzzing or ringing in the ears, called tinnitus (34), can also indicate a hearing loss.

Nearly three-fourths of the test subjects chose 31 as a correct answer:
31.   Someone tells them they talk too loud.
       [This doesn't necessarily mean that they have a hearing problem. A loud   ]
       [voice may be normal for some people.   ]
If someone talks too loud, it could be because they have a hearing loss. However, it could also be that the person's voice is normally loud.

Question H – The correct answers are 36, 37, and 38. Loud noise in modern society has become common, and we often accept it without concern. We should become familiar with simple techniques for judging if noise is too loud, particularly in the workplace, but away from it as well. Any noise that causes pain in the ears (36) is too loud. A good practice at drill sites is the 2-foot rule. Noise is too loud if you can't hear someone who is standing 2 feet away talking to you (37). From any reasonably close distance, however, if you must shout to be heard, then the surrounding noise is too loud (38).

Question I – The correct answers are 40, 41, 42, and 44. Certain administrative controls that conform to company policy and, with respect to exposure time, to current OSHA noise standards can be used to deal with loud noise around the drill rig. For example, individual time spent in high noise areas can be reduced by rotating workers in and out of noisy locations and by telling workers not to linger around the running drill head or compressor areas during lulls in work activity (40). Implementing certain engineering controls may help to reduce drill rig noise levels (41). Examples of the latter may include mufflers and reduced machine vibration.

Workers need to protect the hearing they have left. Some workers feel that because they already have a hearing loss there is no need to protect themselves from loud noises anymore. But some hearing is better than none at all. Based on responses from the test subjects, a high percentage of workers understand that hearing protection is important. Yet, knowing about hearing protection (42) and paying attention to warning signs (44) doesn't always translate into action. However, recognition of ways to protect hearing is a good beginning.

Question J – The correct answers are 45, 46, 47, and 49. Earmuffs and foam earplugs that are not worn correctly will offer very little hearing protection or possibly none at all. Workers who are not aware of the fact that either type of hearing protection can be used incorrectly risk even greater damage to their hearing. Why? Because they will delay leaving noisy work areas since they think their hearing is being protected. Of course, the latter is true only if their earmuffs and earplugs are being used properly.

About half of the test subjects chose 45 as a correct answer:

45. Keep beards or long sideburns trimmed so they don't affect the seal of earmuffs.
    [Correct. Any growth of beard or sideburns will affect the seal and is   ]
    [discouraged.   ]

This means that about half of the test sample were unaware that long sideburns and full beards interfere with the seal of earmuffs. Earmuffs require a good seal around the ear in order to be effective. The pads should be flexible and soft and be capable of adjusting to a comfortable tension. Workers with long hair need to be especially careful.

Rolling and squeezing foam ear plugs (46) is the only way to get them thin enough for proper placement in the ear canal. Pulling the ear **up** and **back** (47) is important because this straightens out the ear canal so that the foam plug can be placed in far enough to be effective.

More than 80% of the test subjects incorrectly chose 48 as a correct answer:

48. After placing the rolled and squeezed ear plug in your ear, release it. It will expand to give you a snug fit.
    [You need to use your finger to keep it in place in the ear canal while it   ]
    [swells up.   ]

A rolled and squeezed foam ear plug will not stay in the ear canal after it expands unless it is held in place with a finger. Holding the plug in the ear for about 20 seconds will allow the plug to expand in place and provide a snug fit.

Both earmuffs and foam plugs should be worn together for extremely loud noise (49). But a worker may be unable to hear any shouts or warnings from other persons. This is a safety hazard. The best way to deal with extremely loud noise is with caution and by combining plugs and muffs only if absolutely necessary.

Finally, dirty ear plugs can cause infection. Hands should be clean to reduce that possibility. Because foam ear plugs are inexpensive, dirty ones should be thrown away and not reused (50).

Question K – The correct answers are 51, 52, 53, and 54. With good hearing, workers will be able to work more safely on the job (51), communicate with other employees, and still be able to hear equipment warning signals and instructions from coworkers. The ability to hear is also a factor in the total enjoyment of family and friends (52). Communicating with others (53) is frustrating and difficult for anyone who has a hearing loss. People must understand that once hearing is lost, it is gone forever (54).

Many people think that hearing aids restore hearing to normal. Hearing aids are simply tiny electrical amplifiers that make all sounds louder. They expand the range of sounds a person can hear, but do nothing for returning the ability to hear. Surgery to rebuild the inner ear and cochlear implants are available, but these are not effective for everyone and they are expensive. The best ways to protect hearing are using hearing protection, limiting time in noisy work areas in accordance with company and OSHA guidelines, and avoiding activities in which exposure is possible.

Scoring Key

The correct answers are marked with an asterisk.[7]

Question   Answer Number

A	1	2	3	4*		
B	5	6	7*	8	9	
C	10	11*	12*	13*		
D	14	15*	16*	17*	18	
E	19	20	21	22*		
F	23*	24	25*	26*	27	28*	29
G	30*	31	32*	33*	34*	35*
H	36*	37*	38*			
I	39	40*	41*	42*	43	44*
J	45*	46*	47*	48	49*	50
K	51*	52*	53*	54*		

---

[7]This page is printed in large type so that it may be copied and used as an overhead transparency.

Summary of Field Test Results

NIOSH evaluated the *Drill Rig Incident* exercise to determine its effectiveness for teaching workers about noise, hearing loss, and hearing protection. A sample of 180 persons participated in a field experiment that consisted of two parts. In the first part, subjects completed either a pretest <u>before</u> working the DRI exercise or a posttest <u>after</u> working the exercise. *Important:* This was an either/or situation, as no subjects completed both a pretest and a posttest. The second part of the experiment consisted of all subjects answering questions (called a self-reporting measure) on their opinion of the validity and utility of the exercise.

The experimental procedure used in the first part is called a "split-group" pretest/posttest assessment. This means that each of the 180 subjects in the sample group was placed, by random draw, into either a control group or an experimental group. The subjects in the control group took the pretest before working the DRI training exercise, and the subjects in the experimental group took the posttest after working the exercise. The dependent variable in the experiment was subjects' score on either the pretest or posttest. The pretest and posttest are an identical set of 24 true or false questions about the topics included in DRI, namely, noise, hearing loss, and hearing protection.

If the experimental group's average score in the posttest would be higher than the control group's average score in the pretest, it would support the belief that subjects in the experimental group learned about noise, hearing loss, and hearing protection from working the DRI exercise and therefore scored higher in the posttest. Those who took the pretest did not have the benefit of working DRI before being tested, so theoretically they know less about noise, etc., and therefore should score lower. If posttest scores are higher than pretest scores, it can be concluded that DRI is the reason and, as a result, it is an effective training exercise.

In this type of investigation, it is important that the experimental and control groups are "equivalent." Equivalent groups, for research purposes, means that subjects have equivalent backgrounds and work-related experience, as well as similar knowledge of the training material content, coming into the experiment. It follows that if the research groups are equivalent, then improved scores in the posttest will be a direct result of the DRI training received and not due to other outside effects.

It was determined that both groups in this experiment are equivalent. The rationale for this is: (1) the groups are statistically large enough so that background knowledge of noise and hearing protection should be about the same, regardless of how much (or how little) is known, (2) subjects were placed into either group by random draw, and (3) their demographics suggest equivalency in terms of age and drilling experience.

Demographics of Subjects

	Control Group (Pretest)			Experimental Group (Posttest)			
	n	**mean**	**SD**	**n**	**mean**	**SD**	**p-value**
Age	103	42.0	11.6	71	43.5	10.1	0.37
Yrs. of exper.	96	13.3	12.1	96	13.3	10.0	0.98

The *t*-test was used to examine whether the control group pretest scores were significantly different from the experimental group posttest scores. The mean posttest score (20.22) was significantly higher than the mean pretest score (18.87), as shown below.

Analysis of Pretest/Posttest Scores Independent Samples *t*-test

Group	n	Mean	SD	t-value	p-value
Control	108	18.87	2.24		
				4.11	<0.0001
Experimental	72	20.22	2.04		

The second part of the experiment consisted of all subjects indicating their level of agreement or disagreement with the statements shown below. This self-reporting measure was used to assess the validity and utility of DRI as a training exercise.

Think about the exercise you just finished. Circle the number that tells how much you <u>agree</u> or <u>disagree</u> with the statements below.

		Definitely Disagree				Definitely Agree
		1	**2**	**3**	**4**	**5**
1.	This situation could happen at a drill site.	1	2	3	4	5
2.	The exercise will help me remember something important about noise and hearing loss.	1	2	3	4	5
3.	I learned something new from this exercise.	1	2	3	4	5
4.	The exercise took too long to complete.	1	2	3	4	5
5.	I liked working the exercise.	1	2	3	4	5
6.	I will use some of the ideas presented to protect my hearing.	1	2	3	4	5
7.	The way the material was presented is a good way for me to learn.	1	2	3	4	5
8.	The exercise was easy to read.	1	2	3	4	5

The number and percentage of subjects who responded to these statements are shown below.

	Statement	N	Agree, %[8]	Disagree, %
1.	This situation could happen at a drill site.	179	92.2	0.6
2.	The exercise will help me remember something important about noise and hearing loss.	179	88.2	1.1
3.	I learned something new from this exercise.	179	73.3	6.2
4.	The exercise took too long to complete.	179	4.5	76.5
5.	I liked working the exercise.	179	66.5	8.4
6.	I will use some of the ideas presented to protect my hearing.	179	89.4	1.1
7.	The way the material was presented is a good way for me to learn.	179	89.9	2.8
8.	The exercise was easy to read.	179	91.6	1.7

Statements 1, 2, and 3 report on participants' assessment of the validity of DRI. As shown above, 99.2% indicate that the "situation could happen at a drill site," 88.2% agree that DRI will help them "remember something important" about noise and hearing loss, and 73.3% of the subjects indicate they "learned something new" from DRI. Finally, 89.4% of the participants indicate they will "use some of the ideas presented to protect" their hearing.

---

[8] "Agree" is the sum of responses 4 and 5.

Answer Key for Pretest / Posttest Questions

Directions: Circle **T** for True or **F** for False.

1.	It takes years of exposure to loud noise for hearing loss to develop.	T	**F**
2.	It's possible to use foam ear plugs incorrectly.	**T**	F
3.	It's possible to use earmuffs incorrectly.	**T**	F
4.	Hearing loss is preventable.	**T**	F
5.	You can't hear someone talking when you are wearing foam ear plugs.	T	**F**
6.	Foam ear plugs are effective only if they are used properly.	**T**	F
7.	Because drill rigs are so noisy, hearing loss is bound to happen to workers.	T	**F**
8.	Our ears eventually adjust to loud noise.	T	**F**
9.	Persons who talk too loud generally have a hearing loss.	T	**F**
10.	Constant ringing in your ears may be a sign of hearing loss.	**T**	F
11.	To people with a hearing loss, normal conversation can sound like people are mumbling.	**T**	F
12.	If you have to shout to be heard around a drill rig, then noise is too loud.	**T**	F
13.	If you can't talk with someone standing 2 feet away while the drill rig is running, then the noise level is too loud.	**T**	F
14.	After placing rolled and squeezed foam ear plugs into your ear canal, they expand to give you a snug fit.	**T**	F
15.	Dirty foam ear plugs should be thrown away and replaced with clean ones.	**T**	F
16.	If foam ear plugs are not rolled and squeezed, they can still be inserted properly into your ears.	T	**F**
17.	Dirty foam ear plugs work as well as clean ones.	T	**F**
18.	Hearing loss can be reversed.	T	**F**
19.	Pulling your ear up and back is not always necessary before inserting foam ear plugs.	T	**F**
20.	Hearing loss is a health problem, not a safety problem.	T	**F**
21.	Once you have a hearing loss, it is permanent.	**T**	F
22.	If you have a hearing loss, time away from a noisy drill rig will allow your hearing to return.	T	**F**
23.	Wearing a hearing aid will bring your hearing back to normal.	T	**F**
24.	One way to ensure that workers use hearing protection is to post "Hearing Protection Required" signs at the workplace.	T	**F**

The correct answers appear in **bold**.

Appendix A: Problem Booklet

Duplicate this copy of the problem booklet for use in your classes. **Booklets should be printed on only one side of the paper.** Each person in your class should have a problem booklet while he/she is working the exercise. The problem booklets are reusable.

Drill Rig Incident

Problem Booklet

Instructions

Begin by reading the **Background** and **Problem** described on the next page. Then answer each of the questions that follow. Do them one at a time in the order they appear. Don't jump ahead, but you may look back at earlier questions and answers at any time.

Some questions ask you to select as MANY answers that you think are correct. Other questions ask you to select only ONE answer, unless you are told to "Try again." Follow the directions for each question.

After you have selected an answer choice to a question, look for its number on the answer sheet. Rub the developing pen between the brackets of your selection on the answer sheet. Be sure to fill in all of the space between brackets; a message will appear and tell if you are correct.

When you have finished the questions, follow the instructions to determine your score for the exercise.

Background

You are the drill foreman of a three-person drilling crew.

The other members of your crew are Billy, your helper, and Willy, an extra laborer.

You have over 20 years of experience as a driller.

Billy's job is to operate the breakout wrench at the rear of the rotary drill rig.

Billy called in sick this morning. The only person you were able to find to replace him on short notice was your cousin Vinny.

Vinny has 5 years' experience on a drilling crew, but hasn't worked on a drill rig for some time.

Your company has recently hired a safety manager, Rip, who has several years of experience in the drilling industry.

Today is a cool and foggy day.

Your company is drilling a 10-inch-diameter replacement water well for the city. They are using a 10-inch-diameter air hammer with 4½-inch API rods as the drill string.

Problem

Your crew's assignment is to pick up where the night shift left off. The night shift strung 10 rod sections plus a dummy casing section in the hole. You are just starting to remove the 10-foot rod sections.

The drill rig is running. As Vinny goes back for a work glove that he dropped, you remind him to "be sure to step back after you attach the automatic chuck." He then latches the breakout wrench around the first pipe section above the threaded joint. You hesitate so he can step back. Vinny does not step back and the wrench begins to spring back. When you realize what is happening, you shout the word "back" to him, but he doesn't move.

Question A

You see that the pipe is not breaking apart and more pressure is needed. Because of the added pressure, you become alarmed since Vinny has not moved out of the way. You know that the wire rope holding the wrench can break. What should you do first? (Choose only ONE unless you are told to "Try again.")

1. Shout again at Vinny to move back.

2. Get Vinny's attention by waving your arms for him to move back.

3. Do nothing and let the wire rope do its job. Vinny will be OK.

4. Shut down the rig using an emergency stop switch, sometimes called a "kill" switch.

Question B

As you hit the kill switch, the wire rope suddenly snaps. The breakout wrench springs back and strikes Vinny in the chest, knocking him down. You move to help him. Fortunately, Vinny only got the wind knocked out of him. He is embarrassed and insists that you start the drill right away. What should you do? (Choose only ONE unless you are told to "Try again.")

5.   Nothing. Vinny didn't get hurt.

6.   Try to find out why the wire rope broke.

7.   Report the incident to your company safety manager right away.

8.   Try to find whose fault it is that Vinny got hit by the wrench.

9.   Start the drill and go back to work.

Question C

You call the safety manager on your cell phone to report the incident. You tell him that Vinny seems to be OK and you expect work to continue. Rip said he would stop by the drill site around lunchtime today. Your crew continues pulling drill rods from the hole.

Rip arrives at the job site before noon and begins to talk with each of you about the incident. Why is Rip doing this? (Select as MANY as you think are correct.)

10. He is trying to find someone to blame.

11. He wants to learn the details of the incident while it is still fresh in your minds.

12. He is looking for information that can be used in future safety classes.

13. He is looking for ways to improve safety in drilling 10-inch holes.

When you have made your selection(s), do the next question.

Question D

After spending some time with your crew, Rip identified several factors that he believes contributed to the incident. What factors did he identify? (Select as MANY as you think are correct.)

14. Poor visibility/bad weather conditions.

15. Failure to follow accepted work practices.

16. Breakdown in communication.

17. Vinny staying in a dangerous position.

18. Loud drill rig noise.

When you have made your selection(s), do the next question.

Question E

Three factors were identified that contributed to the incident: failure to follow accepted work practices, Vinny staying in a dangerous position, and breakdown in communication. All of these will need to be addressed in order to prevent similar incidents in the future, but Rip believes that the breakdown in communication was the underlying factor that caused the others. He believes it should be addressed first because it has the greatest potential for causing other dangerous situations at a drill site. What do you think is the most likely reason for this communication breakdown between you and Vinny? (Choose only ONE unless you are told to "Try again.")

19. Vinny didn't hear you shouting at him because he was using foam ear plugs.

20. Vinny wasn't paying attention.

21. Vinny figured the wire rope was safe and he didn't need to move back.

22. Vinny has a hearing loss.

Question F

Rip knows that all people who work around drill rigs are exposed to loud noise, and he suspects that Vinny may not be the only one to have a hearing loss. For Rip, hearing loss is a safety issue as well as a health issue.

Because others may have a similar hearing loss, Rip believes that a serious injury or fatality could happen to anybody. He decides to design a training program to teach his employees about noise and hearing. He asks for your thoughts on what basic facts to use for building such a program. What would you tell him? (Select as MANY as you think are correct.)

23.   Hearing loss is permanent.

24.   Our ears will eventually adjust to loud noise.

25.   Hearing loss is not reversible.

26.   Hearing loss is preventable.

27.   Hearing loss can be cured.

28.   Hearing loss causes stress in people.

29.   Hearing loss develops after many years of exposure to loud noise.

When you have made your selection(s), do the next question.

Question G

You think that the training program should teach workers how to recognize signs of hearing loss. You want to suggest ways that they can judge for themselves if their hearing is bad. Which of the following would you recommend that Rip include in the training? (Select as MANY as you think are correct.)

30. They often ask people to repeat what they are saying.

31. Someone tells them they talk too loud.

32. They have trouble hearing normal conversation.

33. They complain about people mumbling.

34. They have constant ringing or buzzing in their ears.

35. Others complain that the TV is too loud.

When you have made your selection(s), do the next question.

Question H

Rip thinks it is important for workers to know when noise levels around them are too loud. Without using noise-measuring instruments, there are ways that a person can tell if noise is too loud. Which of the following could Rip use to get this point across in his training? (Select as MANY as you think are correct.)

36. Noise is too loud if it causes pain in your ears.

37. Noise is too loud if you can't hear someone talking from 2 feet away.

38. If you have to shout to be heard, then the noise is too loud.

When you have made your selection(s), do the next question.

Question I

Next, Rip would like drillers to learn how to deal with loud noise around drill rigs. What can Rip tell them to do to protect their hearing? (Select as MANY as you think are correct.)

39. Use more water around the drill hole.

40. Try to spend shorter periods of time in noisy areas during the shift.

41. Ask their supervisor to do something to reduce the noise level.

42. Wear properly fitted hearing protection.

43. Start up any other equipment located at the drill site in order to drown out the drill rig noise.

44. Comply with all "Hearing Protection Required" warning signs.

When you have made your selection(s), do the next question.

Question J

Hearing protection is a simple way to protect the hearing you have left. Rip is concerned that some workers do not know how to use hearing protection properly. What should be included in the training program to teach this? (Select as MANY as you think are correct.)

45. Keep beards or long sideburns trimmed so they don't affect the seal of earmuffs.

46. Roll and squeeze foam ear plugs before inserting them.

47. Pull your ear <u>up</u> and <u>back</u> to open up your ear canal before inserting ear plugs.

48. After placing the rolled and squeezed ear plug in your ear, release it. It will expand to give you a snug fit.

49. Use earmuffs and foam plugs together for extremely loud noise.

50. If foam ear plugs are dirty, you can still use them.

When you have made your selection(s), do the next question.

Question K

Hearing gets worse with age. However, hearing loss will happen much sooner to drillers who don't protect their hearing. What benefits are there to protecting the hearing you have left? (Select as MANY as you think are correct.)

51. Work can be done more safely.

52. Activities with family and friends may be more enjoyable.

53. Communicating with others will be easier and more rewarding.

54. Once it is lost, hearing is gone forever.

End of Problem

Scoring your performance

1. Count the total number of responses you colored in that were marked "correct." Write this number in the first blank on the answer sheet.

2. Count the total number of "incorrect" responses you colored in. Subtract this number from 21. Write the difference in the second blank on the answer sheet.

3. Add the numbers on the first and second blanks. This is your score.

The highest possible score is 54.

The lowest possible score is 0.

Appendix B: Blank Answer Sheets

Copies of these blank answer sheets may be duplicated in the normal fashion.
However, the answers that are found within the brackets must be printed on these blank
answer sheets in invisible ink. These answers are found in appendix C. If you have the
capability to print invisible ink, make copies of the blank answer sheets. Make a master
of the answers that appear in appendix C. Then print the invisible ink on the blank
answer sheets, making sure that all pages print and that the appropriate answers line
up with the appropriate blanks. The Master Answer Sheet shows all of the answers in
their proper places.

The exercise is designed to be used in small groups. You will need one answer sheet
for each group of three to five persons in your class. The answer sheets are
consumable. You will need a new set for each class.

A special developing pen is needed by the person within each group who marks the
answer sheet. "PENIB" developing pens may be obtained from SICPA Customer
Service, 8000 Research Way, Springfield, VA 22153, phone: 1–888–742–7287.

Answer Sheet for *Drill Rig Incident*

Use this answer sheet to mark your selections. Rub the developing pen gently and smoothly between the brackets. Don't scrub the pen or the message may blur. Be sure to color in the entire message once you have made a selection. Otherwise, you may not get the information you need. The last part of the message will tell you what to do next.

Question A (Choose only ONE unless you are told to "Try again.")

1. [   ]

2. [   ]
    [   ]

3. [   ]
    [   ]

4. [   ]
    [   ]

Question B (Choose only ONE unless you are told to "Try again.")

5. [   ]
    [   ]

6. [   ]
    [   ]

7. [   ]
    [   ]
    [   ]

8. [   ]

9. [   ]

Question C (Select as MANY as you think are correct.)

10. [   ]

11. [   ]
    [   ]

12. [   ]
    [   ]

13. [   ]
    [   ]

Question D (Select as MANY as you think are correct.)

14. [   ]
     [   ]

15. [   ]
     [   ]

16. [   ]

17. [   ]
     [   ]

18. [   ]
     [   ]

Question E (Choose only ONE unless you are told to "Try again.")

19. [   ]
     [   ]

20. [   ]
     [   ]

21. [   ]
     [   ]

22. [   ]
     [   ]

Question F (Select as MANY as you think are correct.)

23. [   ]

24. [   ]
     [   ]

25. [   ]

26. [   ]
     [   ]

27. [   ]
     [   ]

28. [   ]
     [   ]

29. [   ]

Question G (Select as MANY as you think are correct.)

30. [   ]
     [   ]

31. [   ]
     [   ]

32. [   ]

33. [   ]
     [   ]

34. [   ]

35. [   ]

Question H (Select as MANY as you think are correct.)

36. [   ]

37. [   ]
     [   ]

38. [   ]
     [   ]

Question I (Select as MANY as you think are correct.)

39. [   ]

40. [   ]
     [   ]

41. [   ]
     [   ]

42. [   ]

43. [   ]
     [   ]

44. [   ]
     [   ]

Question J (Select as MANY as you think are correct.)

45. [   ]
     [   ]

46. [   ]
     [   ]

47. [   ]
     [   ]

48. [   ]
     [   ]

49. [   ]
     [   ]

50. [   ]
     [   ]
     [   ]

Question K (Select as MANY as you think are correct.)

51. [   ]

52. [   ]

53. [   ]

54. [   ]
     [   ]

Finding your score

Number of "Correct" answers you colored in   = (1)_____

21 minus number of incorrect answers you colored in   = (2)_____

Add (1) and (2) to get your total score   = (3)_____

Highest possible score = 54

Lowest possible score = 0

Appendix C: Invisible Ink Answers

These pages contain the answers that must be printed in the blanks of the answer sheet in appendix B. These answers are spaced and sequenced correctly so that they match up exactly with the appropriate blanks on the answer sheet.

Once the answers have been printed in the answer sheet blanks, the developing pen reveals the formerly invisible printed message.

You may obtain preprinted answer sheets or you may prepare your own copies. To learn more about these options and to determine how many answer sheets and developing pens you will need, see the "Introduction" section at the beginning of this Instructor's Copy.

This is not the first thing that needs to be done. Try again.

This is not the first thing that needs to be done. Besides, you don't want to cause Vinny to look away from the drill. Try again.

You know that wire ropes have been known to snap. You should do something now. Try again.

Correct. You need to stop the rig before Vinny gets hurt. Do the next question.

There was no apparent injury, but for Vinny's sake something should be done. Try again.

This isn't important right now. You will probably learn why the rope broke later on. Try again.

Correct. For Vinny's protection in case any medical problems develop later, the safety manager will need to have some record of the incident. Do the next question.

Finding someone to blame is not important. Try again.

You need to do something else first. Try again.

Finding someone to blame isn't going to help the situation.

Correct. Since no one got hurt he wants to learn the details before anyone forgets what happened.

Correct. He may be able to prevent similar incidents by developing SOPs and safety or toolbox meetings using this information.

Correct. It is often possible to develop safer ways to complete a task by looking at details of previous incidents.

Even though the weather was foggy, the distance between you and Vinny was so close that visibility was not a problem.

Correct. The usual work practice is for your helper to back away as soon as he puts the wrench on a rod section.

Correct. This is an obvious factor that led to the incident.

Correct. He stayed there because he didn't follow your directions to move back.

Even though drill rigs are noisy, Vinny should have been able to hear your directions.

Vinny would have been able to hear you shouting even if he was wearing foam ear plugs. Try again.

Vinny knows the dangers in drilling, so he was probably paying very close attention. Try again.

Vinny has enough experience around drill rigs to know that wire ropes can break. Try again.

Correct. If Vinny has a hearing loss, this would explain why he didn't hear your original instructions or your shouting. Do the next question.

Correct. Once your hearing is lost, it will never come back.

Our ears don't adjust to loud noise; we just lose our ability to hear normal sounds.

Correct. Damage to a person's hearing cannot be reversed.

Correct. There are a number of things a person can do to prevent hearing loss.

There is no way to "cure" hearing loss. Hearing aids can help some people, but not everyone can be helped by a hearing aid.

Correct. Stress can develop in persons who have lost some of their hearing because communication becomes difficult.

Permanent hearing loss can develop very quickly If noise levels are high.

Correct. If this happens most of the time, it's one sign that a person may have a hearing loss.

This doesn't necessarily mean that they have a hearing problem. A loud voice may be normal for some people.

Correct. In most cases, this indicates a hearing loss.

Correct. With a hearing loss, it is difficult to hear all of the sounds that are spoken. Conversation may sound like people are mumbling.

Correct. Called tinnitus, this is a classic symptom of hearing loss.

Correct.

Correct. Loud noise often causes physical pain in a person's ears.

Correct. Some call this the "2-foot rule," and it's a good way for drillers and other workers to realize that noise in their workplace is too loud.

Correct. Noise is too loud if you can't hear someone talking from 2 feet away

This will not contribute to noise reduction.

Correct. Getting away from drill rig noise for short periods of time will help to reduce their total exposure time during a shift.

Correct. It's possible that some type of control can be used to reduce drill rig noise levels or time of worker exposure to noise.

Correct. This is a sure way to protect a person's hearing.

Noise from other equipment just adds to the total noise level and would only make matters worse.

Correct. This is a reminder to all workers that noise levels are high and that everyone should be using hearing protection.

Correct. Any growth of beard or sideburns will affect the seal and is discouraged.

Correct. This makes the ear plugs thinner so they can be inserted into your ear canal.

Correct. This will straighten out the ear canal and make it easier to insert the plug.

You need to use your finger to keep it in place in the ear canal while it swells up.

Correct. Combining both types of hearing protection should be done <u>only</u> for very loud noise.

Dirty ear plugs do not give the same protection as clean ones. There is also a danger of infection. Dirty ear plugs should be thrown away and replaced with new ones.

Correct.

Correct.

Correct.

Correct. Although hearing aids may help, they can never bring back normal hearing.

Appendix D: Pretest / Posttest Questions

This page contains the pretest / posttest questions that may be administered to the class. Duplicate these for each person in your class. **These should be printed on only one side of the paper.**

Pretest / Posttest Questions

Directions: Circle **T** for True or **F** for False.

1.	It takes years of exposure to loud noise for hearing loss to develop.	T	F
2.	It's possible to use foam ear plugs incorrectly.	T	F
3.	It's possible to use earmuffs incorrectly.	T	F
4.	Hearing loss is preventable.	T	F
5.	You can't hear someone talking when you are wearing foam ear plugs.	T	F
6.	Foam ear plugs are effective only if they are used properly.	T	F
7.	Because drill rigs are so noisy, hearing loss is bound to happen to workers.	T	F
8.	Our ears eventually adjust to loud noise.	T	F
9.	Persons who talk too loud generally have a hearing loss.	T	F
10.	Constant ringing in your ears may be a sign of hearing loss.	T	F
11.	To people with a hearing loss, normal conversation can sound like people are mumbling.	T	F
12.	If you have to shout to be heard around a drill rig, then noise is too loud.	T	F
13.	If you can't talk with someone standing 2 feet away while the drill rig is running, then the noise level is too loud.	T	F
14.	After placing rolled and squeezed foam ear plugs into your ear canal, they expand to give you a snug fit.	T	F
15.	Dirty foam ear plugs should be thrown away and replaced with clean ones.	T	F
16.	If foam ear plugs are not rolled and squeezed, they can still be inserted properly into your ears.	T	F
17.	Dirty foam ear plugs work as well as clean ones.	T	F
18.	Hearing loss can be reversed.	T	F
19.	Pulling your ear up and back is not always necessary before inserting foam ear plugs.	T	F
20.	Hearing loss is a health problem, not a safety problem.	T	F
21.	Once you have a hearing loss, it is permanent.	T	F
22.	If you have a hearing loss, time away from a noisy drill rig will allow your hearing to return.	T	F
23.	Wearing a hearing aid will bring your hearing back to normal.	T	F
24.	One way to ensure that workers use hearing protection is to post "Hearing Protection Required" signs at the workplace.	T	F